Lymphatic Drainage Massage

The Complete Guide to Understanding and Performing Lymphatic Drainage Massage Yourself at Home

Dani Twain

Copyright Notice

All rights reserved. No part of this publication may be reproduced, stored in a retrieval system or transmitted in any form or by any means, including electronic, digital, mechanical, photocopying, audio recording, printing or otherwise, without written permission from the publisher or the author.

Contents

COPYRIGHT

INTRODUCTION

Chapter 1: What is Lymphatic Drainage Massage?

Chapter 2: Types of Lymphatic Drainage Massage

Chapter 3: How to Perform Lymphatic Drainage Yourself

Chapter 4: General Principles of Massage

Lower Body Massage Techniques

Upper Body Massage Techniques

CHAPTER 5

The Power of Lymph Drainage Massage for Your Face and Neck

How Lymphatic Drainage Massage Works

How to Incorporate Lymphatic Drainage Massage into Your Routine

Lymphatic Drainage Massage of the Chest

Lymphatic Drainage Massage of the Abdomen

Lymphatic Drainage Back Massage

Lymphatic Drainage Hand Massage

Chapter 6: Techniques for Performing Lymphatic Drainage Foot Massage at Home

Chapter 7: Lymphatic Drainage Massage Techniques

Suitability of Lymphatic Drainage Massage

Differences and Advantages Over Other Massage Types

Chapter 8: Benefits of Lymphatic Drainage

Chapter 9: How Lifestyle Affects the Lymphatic System

Chapter 10: After a Lymphatic Drainage Massage

Chapter 11: Other Types of Massages Supporting Lymphatic Drainage

Chapter 12: Contraindications to Lymphatic Drainage

Conclusion

Introduction

Do you ever feel like your legs are heavy, or notice varicose veins, stretch marks, cellulite, or water retention? These can all be signs of a damaged lymphatic system. While there are professional treatments available, you can also take steps to drain your lymphatic system at home through self-massage.

Lymphatic drainage is a massage technique that helps move lymph fluid through your body. Usually, a trained therapist performs this technique, but you can also learn to do it yourself at home.

This technique was developed in the 1930s by a Danish doctor named Emil Vodder. Over time, the Vodder method has been improved through teaching and scientific studies.

What are the basics of lymphatic drainage? What benefits does it offer? How can you perform lymphatic drainage at home, and what precautions should you take? Here's everything you need to know about practicing lymphatic drainage safely at home.

Chapter 1

What is Lymphatic Drainage Massage?

Lymphatic drainage massage is a way to help move lymph fluid through your body, either using special equipment or your hands. This massage not only improves how your body looks but also has health benefits.

The key to this massage is focusing on specific areas of your body, not just warming up muscles. A therapist or practitioner moves their hands along the lines where lymph flows, helping to get the fluid moving.

How Does Lymph Flow Work?

The lymphatic system is a natural part of your body that helps remove waste and excess fluid. It can pump out about 2-4 liters of waste and fluid every day. However, when you get older, your lymph flow can slow down, and poor diet can also cause problems.

When the lymphatic system doesn't work well, fluid builds up in your body, and lymph nodes get clogged with waste and toxins. This can disrupt your metabolism and weaken your immune system, making you more likely to get sick.

To avoid these issues, it's important to keep your lymphatic system working well. You can help by learning and practicing lymphatic drainage at home.

Chapter 2

Types of Lymphatic Drainage Massage

There are two main types of lymphatic drainage massage: manual and mechanical.

Manual Lymphatic Drainage Massage

This type of massage is done by a specialist using their hands. With smooth, rhythmic movements, the therapist massages the lymph nodes to increase lymph flow. To help you relax even more, they might use aromatic oils that have a calming effect during the massage.

Mechanical Lymphatic Drainage Massage

This method uses special equipment to perform the massage. The equipment uses electrical impulses to activate nerve endings and improve lymph flow. Mechanical massage not only helps remove excess fluid from the lymphatic system but also improves blood flow and muscle function. This boosts cellular metabolism, leading to a firmer body, healthier skin, better overall well-being, and stronger immunity. The main types of mechanical lymphatic drainage massage are:

- LPG (Endermology or Vacuum Roller): Uses rollers to massage the skin and stimulate lymph flow.

- Galvanization: Uses a mild electric current to stimulate lymph nodes.
- Electrophoresis: Uses electric currents to push medication into the skin, enhancing lymph flow.
- Pressotherapy: Uses air pressure to massage the body and improve lymph circulation.
- Microcurrent Drainage: Uses low-level electrical currents to stimulate lymph flow.

Massage Areas

Lymphatic drainage body massage can target different areas, including:

- Legs
- Arms
- Back
- Abdomen
- Neck

These treatments can help improve lymph flow and reduce swelling in specific parts of the body.

Chapter 3

How to Perform Lymphatic Drainage Yourself

You can perform a lymphatic drainage self-massage by following these simple steps:

Preparation

1. Find a Comfortable Space: Choose a quiet, comfortable place where you can lie down or sit comfortably during the massage.
2. Elevate Your Legs: Place a pillow or cushion under your ankles to promote lymphatic return.

Steps to Follow

1. Diaphragmatic Breathing

- Hand Positioning: Place your hands below your chest, under your ribs.

- Breathing Exercise: Take a deep breath through your nose to open your diaphragm, then exhale deeply through your mouth to release tension. This helps with oxygen transport and lymphatic stimulation. Repeat this exercise 3 times.

2. Neck Massage

- Finger Placement: Use the index and middle fingers of both hands.

- Massage Movement: Make gentle circular movements over the lymph nodes on either side of your neck, above the collarbones. Do this 15 times, counterclockwise.

3. Armpit Massage

- Hand Placement: Place one hand in the opposite armpit and stretch upwards and forwards.
- Repetitions: Repeat 15 times, then switch to the other side.

4. Groin Massage

- Hand Placement: Place one hand in the hollow of your groin, gently pressing your fingers into the skin.
- Massage Movement: Make gentle movements towards your navel. Repeat 15 times to stimulate lymphatic drainage in the pelvic area.

5. Chest Massage

- Seated Position: Sit comfortably.
- Massage Movements:
  - Slide both hands from your waist towards your armpits. Repeat 5 times.

- Then slide your hands from your groin towards your armpits. Repeat 5 times.

6. Leg Massage
- Seated Position: Raise one leg on a stool.
- Massage Movements: Using slow, light movements, gently massage your legs from your ankles to your thighs, both on the outer and inner sides. Repeat 5 times, then switch to the other leg.

7. Arm Massage
- Massage Movements: Use gentle, even pressure to massage your arms from your hands to your shoulders, then towards your groin.

8. Face and Neck Massage

- Neck Massage: Lightly massage the back of your neck with your hands, head slightly forward. Do this 15 times.

- Jaw Massage: Starting from the front of your ears, use your fingertips to massage your jaw towards your chin.

- Neck to Armpit: Slide your hand from the front of your neck to your armpit. Repeat this 5 times.

9. Final Steps

- Clear Lymph Nodes: Repeat the lymph node clearing steps for the neck (step 2), armpits (step 3), groin (step 4), and diaphragm (step 1) to return to normal breathing.

- Hydrate: Drink plenty of water after the session to help flush out waste.

Chapter 4

General Principles of Massage

Massages should only affect the skin with gentle pressure. Never press too hard and keep your hands relaxed. Do not massage swollen or infected areas.

Do not use lotions or other products, only your hands.

It is important to hydrate well, ideally drinking 2 to 4 glasses of water after each massage to help cleanse the body.

You can also use lymphatic drainage boots to enjoy a massage at home whenever you want.

Preparation Before the Massage
These methods help stimulate the lymphatic system and prepare the lymph nodes to absorb more fluid.

1. Lymphatic Breathing
Deep breathing helps circulate the fluid through the vessels and lymph nodes.

- Hand Positioning: Place both hands on your ribs.
- Breathing Exercise: Breathe slowly and deeply, feeling the air move towards your abdomen. Slowly exhale through your mouth. Perform this operation 10 times in a row, pausing after each series.

2. Massage the Front of the Neck

- Finger Placement: Place the index and middle fingers of each hand on either side of your neck, just below the earlobe.
- Massage Movement: Stretch the skin by gently sliding your fingers towards your shoulders, then release. Repeat 5 times. Move your hands down and repeat until you have massaged the entire neck.

3. Massage the Side of the Neck

- Hand Placement: Place the palm of each hand on either side of your neck, under the ears.
- Massage Movement: Slowly move both hands down and back.

4. Massage the Back of the Neck

- Hand Placement: Place the palms of your hands on the back of your neck, near the hairline.

- Massage Movement: Gently slide your hands down the neck toward the spine.

5. Massage the Underside of the Arms

- Caution: Do not perform this movement on areas that have been treated following surgery or other operations.

- Hand Placement: Place the palm of your hand under your armpit.

- Massage Movement: Gently pump the palm up and toward the body. Repeat on the other arm.

6. Massage Behind the Knees

- Hand Placement: Place both hands behind the knee so that your fingers point toward each other.

- Massage Movement: Gently press and roll your hands upward on the back of your knee. Repeat on the other knee.

Upper Body Massage Techniques

Use these techniques to help drain lymphatic fluid from the chest, shoulder, and arm.

To Massage the Chest

- Hand Placement: Place the palm of your hand flat on the opposite side of your chest, slightly above the breast.

- Massage Movement: Move your hand up to the chest and over the collarbone.

Continue towards the neck until the skin covering the chest is taut, then release.

To Massage the Shoulder
- Arm Position: Place your arm on a table or armrest.
- Hand Placement: Place the other hand on the shoulder of the resting arm.
- Massage Movement: Run your hand over the back of the shoulder and towards the neck.

To Massage the Upper Arm
- Arm Position: Place your arm on a table or armrest.
- Finger Placement: Place the two middle fingers of the other hand on the inside of your arm, under the shoulder.
- Massage Movement: Gently slide your fingers outward from the arm. Wrap your

hand around the outside of your upper arm and bring your hand towards the inside of your arm.

To Massage the Entire Arm
- Starting Position: Start at the shoulder.
- Hand Movement: Use the palm of your hand to stretch the skin upward. Lower your hand toward the upper arm and stretch the skin toward the shoulder. Continue moving down the arm, always moving the skin upwards. Stop at the wrist.

To Massage the Fingers
- Starting Position: Start at the base of the swollen finger, near the palm.
- Hand Movement: Use your index finger and thumb to stretch the skin from the finger toward the hand. Continue this movement

across the entire finger. Remember to direct the fluid toward your hand.

Lower Body Massage Techniques
Start the massage at the top of your leg and work down to your foot. Use a pillow or stool for support.

To Massage the Upper Leg
- Starting Position: Start at the top of your leg.
- Hand Placement: Place one hand on the opposite inner thigh, near the groin, and the other hand on your buttock.
- Massage Movement: Gently tighten the skin by moving your hand from the inner thigh to the outer thigh and upwards. Move your hands further down the leg and repeat the stretching movement. Stop above the knee.

To Massage the Lower Leg

- Starting Position: Start just below the knee.
- Hand Placement: Place one hand on the shin and the other on the back of the calf.
- Massage Movement: Gently stretch the skin upwards. Continue this movement down toward the ankle and top of the foot. Always make upward movements.

To Massage the Toes

- Hand Placement: Use your thumb and index finger to stroke the skin from the tip of each toe toward the base.

Chapter 5

The Power of Lymph Drainage Massage for Your Face and Neck

Lymphatic drainage massage for the face and neck offers many benefits, such as a more defined facial contour, reduced double chin, less dark circles under the eyes, reduced swelling, and improved skin condition. Regularly practicing this massage can help even out your skin tone and remove toxins from your body.

What if I told you there's a massage technique you can easily add to your daily skincare routine? It helps reduce puffiness, dullness, stress-related skin problems, and overall improves your skin's appearance. It's called lymphatic drainage massage. You can either book a session with a massage therapist or learn to do it yourself at home while applying your skincare products.

How Lymphatic Drainage Massage Works

Lymph fluid, a clear liquid, is collected and transported by lymphatic vessels. Unlike the circulatory system, which is propelled by the heart, the lymphatic system relies on muscle movement and body activity to move fluid. Lymphatic drainage massage helps by gently manipulating the lymphatic vessels, aiding fluid movement and drainage. This technique helps eliminate waste products, toxins, and excess fluids from your tissues, promoting a healthy complexion.

Lymphatic drainage massage has been used for centuries in practices like Ayurveda and Traditional Chinese Medicine (TCM). I've recently started doing it daily and noticed less tenderness and puffiness around my jaw and neck.

How to Incorporate Lymphatic Drainage Massage into Your Routine

Face and neck lymphatic drainage massage is generally safe, but if you have health concerns, consult a trained professional and always be gentle. Follow these steps to get started on your own:

1. Apply Face Oil or Balm: Start by applying a face oil or balm to your face.

2. Warm Up Your Neck and Head: Gently massage the base of your neck, where it meets your shoulders, using circular motions.

3. Forehead Massage: Use light pressure strokes to massage your forehead from the center towards the temples.

4. Under-Eye Massage: With two knuckles, stroke from under your eyes along the cheekbones towards the temples.

5. Ear Massage: Massage the areas in front and behind your ears using circular motions.

6. Jawline Massage: Stroke your jawline from the center of your chin towards your

ears to promote lymphatic flow in the lower face.

7. Neck Massage: Stroke down the sides of your neck towards your collarbone, starting from underneath each ear.

8. Repeat: Perform the above steps on both sides of your head and neck, maintaining a slow, rhythmic pace throughout.

9. Hydrate: Drink plenty of water after the massage to support the lymphatic system.

You can incorporate this massage at any stage of your skincare routine. Try doing it when applying your cleansing balm, beeswax balm, or face oil. Enjoy the benefits of a lymphatic drainage massage!

Lymphatic Drainage Massage of the Chest

Many women are concerned about the shape and appearance of their breasts, especially during breastfeeding and motherhood when the body goes through noticeable changes. A properly performed lymphatic drainage massage of the chest can help improve the elasticity of the muscle frame, fight loss of tone and age-related changes, improve skin condition, and prevent the formation of tumors.

Steps for a Lymphatic Drainage Massage

How do you start lymphatic drainage massage? Begin with deep breathing. Breathing helps stimulate your lymphatic system throughout your entire body. As you go through these steps, remember to keep breathing deeply.

Step 1: Clear Your Lymph Nodes

- Apply Oil: After showering or before bed, apply a few drops of breast oil to your hand and place them under your breast.

- Stimulate Lymph Nodes: Place your palm inside your armpit with your thumb on the outside and gently pump upwards into your armpit. Repeat 5-10 times on each side.

Step 2: Massage Your Breasts

- Under-Breast Massage: Place your palm under your breast and massage along the bra line, up and into your armpits. Repeat three times on each side.

- Over-Breast Massage: Place your palm over your breastbone in the center of your chest. Imagine drawing a rainbow with your fingers towards your armpits while gently massaging your breasts with your whole hand.

- Collarbone Massage: Place the palm of one hand below your breast and gently hold it. Using the palm of the other hand, massage your breast towards your collarbone.

Step 3: Shake Your Breasts, Freestyle

Feel comfortable and have fun! One option is to hold a breast with both hands and give it a little jiggle, or pump inwards towards the chest bone. Repeat on both breasts. Alternatively, hold your breasts with both hands and pump them inwards in circular motions while rotating your shoulders.

Step 4: Send Love to Your Breasts and Your Heart

Hug your breasts with both hands. Close your eyes and take a deep breath. As you inhale, imagine sending a majestic rainbow and love into your heart. As you exhale, imagine releasing a grey cloud of any residual feelings of stress or emotional pain. This is where your heart chakra is, so treat it with self-love and acceptance.

Lymphatic Drainage Massage of the Abdomen

Lymphatic drainage massage of the abdomen uses light fingertip movements. This massage technique can boost immunity, help remove toxins, improve lymphatic drainage, reduce swelling, and even help with weight loss and body shaping.

Session Duration

The duration of a lymphatic drainage session can vary:

- Professional Session: A session with a qualified practitioner usually lasts between 30 and 60 minutes, depending on the treatment goals and methods used.
- Self-Massage at Home: If you're doing the massage yourself, it can take between 10

and 20 minutes, depending on your comfort and needs.

Best Practices for Lymphatic Drainage Self-Massage

While self-massage is not a substitute for professional treatment, it can help improve lymphatic circulation at home. Here are some best practices:

1. Create a Calm Environment: Make sure you are relaxed in a quiet space. You can lie down on a comfortable bed or a yoga mat.
2. Use Light Pressure: The lymphatic system is close to the skin's surface, so gentle pressure is enough. Movements should be gentle and relaxing, not painful.
3. Start with the Lymph Nodes: Begin by gently massaging the lymph nodes in your

groin and armpits with circular motions to stimulate them.

4. Drainage Movements: After stimulating the lymph nodes, move to your abdomen. Use gentle, circular sweeping motions toward the lymph nodes in your groin. Start on the right side of your stomach, as most lymph from the digestive system drains to the chest duct on the right. Always move towards the lymph nodes to encourage lymph flow.

5. Breathe Deeply: Deep breathing can help stimulate lymphatic flow. Try to synchronize your breathing with your massage movements for maximum relaxation.

6. Take Your Time: Don't rush. Take your time massaging each area, focusing on tight or swollen spots.

7. Hydrate: Drink plenty of water (at least 1.5 liters per day) after your session to help eliminate toxins.

Key Drainage Points on the Abdomen

Lymphatic drainage of the abdomen targets the lymphatic vessels and nodes in the abdomen and pelvic region, particularly focusing on:

- Inguinal Lymph Nodes: Located in the groin, these nodes drain lymph from the lower parts of the trunk, including part of the abdomen and pelvis.
- Stomach Lymphatic Vessels: These vessels run along the surface of the abdomen and help collect lymph from this area.

Lymphatic Drainage Back Massage

Lymphatic drainage back massage can speed up lymph flow, improve overall well-being, reduce tension and swelling, and even help with fat reduction. Back or lumbar pain is one of the most common complaints among people of all ages, especially those who are active or elderly.

Benefits of Lymphatic Drainage Massage
Causes and Types of Back Pain

Back pain can be caused by various factors, including poor posture, muscle tension, lack of physical activity, and more. The nature of the pain can vary and will determine the best treatment. Back pain can be classified by its duration:

- Acute Pain: Lasts up to 6 weeks.

- Subacute Pain: Lasts between 6 to 12 weeks.

- Chronic Pain: Lasts more than 12 weeks, sometimes even a lifetime.

Back pain can feel dull, throbbing, sharp, sudden, or spreading to other areas like the legs. The intensity can range from mild to severe.

Common Causes of Back Pain

1. Irregular Posture: Sitting or standing with poor posture can lead to back pain over time.

2. Sports Injuries: Active sports can cause back pain due to injuries or improper exercise techniques.

3. Heavy Lifting: Lifting heavy items improperly can cause back pain. Always squat to lift heavy objects.

4. Spinal Diseases: Conditions like scoliosis, lordosis, and osteochondrosis can cause back pain.

5. Menstruation: Women may experience lower back pain during menstruation due to nerve impulses from the ovaries and uterus.

6. Pregnancy: In the last months of pregnancy, back pain is common due to changes in balance.

Treatment of Back Pain

The treatment depends on the cause and duration of the pain:

- Acute Pain: Treated with muscle relaxants, anti-inflammatory medicines, painkillers, and sometimes heat or cold therapy, massages, or water treatments. In some cases, spinal injections or surgery might be needed.

- Chronic Pain: Managed with regular exercise, massages, and other physiotherapy procedures.

Massage Therapy Benefits

Massage therapy helps improve overall health and wellness, with specific benefits including:

- Improves Circulation and Lymphatic System Function: Enhances immune function.
- Relieves Stress and Anxiety: Promotes relaxation.
- Promotes Joint Mobility and Flexibility: Enhances movement and reduces stiffness.

- Reduces Muscle Pain and Tension: Eases discomfort.
- Stimulates the Nervous System: Increases body awareness.
- Softens Scar Tissue: Improves skin and tissue health.

Lymphatic Drainage Massage

Lymphatic drainage massage is especially effective for preventing diseases, improving blood circulation, and treating lymphatic system disorders. Many people today have a disrupted lymphatic system due to lack of movement, sedentary work, tight clothing, poor diet, and harmful habits. The more causes there are, the faster the lymph flow is disrupted.

By incorporating lymphatic drainage massage into your routine, you can support your lymphatic system, enhance your immune function, and improve your overall health.

Lymphatic Drainage Hand Massage

Performing lymphatic drainage hand massage regularly can greatly benefit your skin, remove toxins from your body, boost lymph flow, and reduce swelling and unwanted fat deposits quickly.

Benefits of Lymphatic Drainage Hand Massage

Lymphatic drainage hand massage helps improve overall health and rejuvenate the body. It can be done manually or with special equipment.

Types of Lymphatic Drainage Hand Massage

1. Manual Massage: This depends on the goals:

 - Surface: For face and neck, healing and relaxing effects.

 - Deep: Targets cellulite and fat layers, eliminates excess water.

 - Point (Therapeutic): Focuses on lymph nodes.

 - Mainline: Treats the entire body's lymphatic system.

2. Hardware Massage: Uses special devices like:

 - Pressotherapy: Uses compressed air to reduce volume in hips, arms, and legs.

 - Microcurrent Drainage: Uses pulsed current to accelerate fluid movement.

 - Vacuum: Deeply treats all body areas.

Indications and Contraindications

Indications:
- Muscle weakness and numbness.
- Sagging hand skin.
- Excess fat.
- Weak immune system.
- Poor blood circulation.
- Swollen hands.
- Chronic lymphostasis, and more.

Contraindications:
- Diabetes.
- Cardiovascular diseases.
- Bleeding disorders.
- Cancer.
- Thrombophlebitis.
- Skin diseases.
- Lymphadenitis and lymphadenopathy.

- Neuralgia.

- Skin damage or inflammation.

Note: Consult a doctor before undergoing lymphatic drainage hand massage during pregnancy.

Effects of Lymphatic Drainage Hand Massage

When performed correctly, lymphatic drainage hand massage achieves several benefits:

- Removes lymph stagnation.
- Increases deep muscle tone.
- Improves metabolism.
- Reduces subcutaneous fat.
- Relieves muscle spasms.

Rules for Lymphatic Drainage Hand Massage

To achieve these effects, follow these guidelines:

- Wait at least 2 hours after eating before a massage.

- Drink at least 2 liters of water during the course.

- Use gentle, wave-like movements along lymph flow lines.

- Avoid applying strong pressure.

- Finish with a contrast shower.

- Massage duration should be between 30 minutes to an hour.

- Rest for at least 30 minutes after the massage.

Performing Lymphatic Drainage Hand Massage at Home

You can perform manual lymphatic drainage hand massage at home, especially beneficial after breast surgery. Follow these steps:

1. Extend your hand in front of you.
2. Use circular patting movements from wrist to elbow, repeat 10 times on each hand.
3. Stroke the axillary and elbow areas smoothly.
4. End by stroking from fingertip to wrist on the palms, repeat 10 times.
5. Rest for at least 30 minutes afterward.

Note: Even with correct technique at home, professional massage sessions offer comprehensive benefits.

Lymphatic drainage hand massage is a beneficial practice for improving health and maintaining well-being, whether performed professionally or at home.

Lymphatic Drainage Foot Massage

Performing lymphatic drainage foot massage correctly can greatly improve skin condition, tighten buttocks, shape the figure, and alleviate issues like spider veins, heaviness, swelling, varicose veins, and excess weight.

Benefits of Lymphatic Drainage Foot Massage

Lymphatic drainage massage of the legs not only restores lymph movement but also brings about several other positive effects:

- Blood Capillaries: Strengthen and expand, creating new channels for blood flow.

- Skin: Speeds up metabolic processes, activates tissue nutrition (trophism), enhances collagen and elastin production, and loosens sticky protein fibers.

- Subcutaneous Fat: Melts fat and softens rough connective tissue partitions, reducing cellulite.

- Muscles: Relieves spasms and restores healthy tone.

Effects of Lymphatic Drainage Foot Massage

The results of lymphatic drainage foot massage include:

- Reduction of swelling and extra centimeters.
- Slimmer legs with graceful ankles, fitting into old jeans.

- Improved skin quality, tightened and evened microrelief.

- Reduction and disappearance of stretch marks.

- Erasure of pigment spots.

- Reduction of cellulite ("orange peel").

- Minimization of varicose veins and less noticeable vascular network (avoid massage if veins are bulging or there are lumps).

Additional Benefits

Apart from improving leg health, lymphatic drainage foot massage benefits the entire body by:

- Eliminating toxins.
- Strengthening the immune system.
- Enhancing overall health and well-being.

Indications for Lymphatic Drainage Massage of the Legs

Consider lymphatic drainage massage if you experience:

- General or local swelling of the lower extremities.
- Cellulite.
- Persistent feeling of heaviness in the legs.
- Cold feet sensation.
- Impaired metabolism.
- Body intoxication.

Performing lymphatic drainage foot massage can effectively address these issues and promote better health and vitality.

Lymphatic drainage foot massage offers numerous benefits for improving leg health and overall well-being. Here's what you can expect from this therapeutic technique:

Effects of Lymphatic Drainage Foot Massage

- Reduction of Swelling: Helps eliminate swelling and reduce excess fluid retention.

- Improved Leg Shape: Promotes slimmer legs with toned muscles and graceful ankles, making it easier to fit into old clothes.

- Enhanced Skin Quality: Tightens the skin and evens out its texture, leading to smoother and more even skin.

- Reduction of Stretch Marks: Diminishes and in some cases completely eliminates stretch marks.

- **Reduction of Pigment Spots:** Fades and reduces the appearance of pigment spots on the skin.

- **Cellulite Reduction:** Diminishes the appearance of cellulite, also known as "orange peel" skin.

- **Varicose Veins Management:** Helps manage early signs of varicose veins and makes pronounced vascular networks less noticeable. However, avoid massage if varicose veins are advanced with bulging or lumpy formations.

- **Relief from Leg Discomfort:** Alleviates feelings of heaviness, discomfort, and pain in the legs.

- **Overall Body Benefits:** Assists in detoxifying the body, strengthens the immune system, and contributes to improved health and well-being.

Indications for Lymphatic Drainage Massage of the Legs

Consider lymphatic drainage foot massage if you experience:

- General or local swelling of the lower extremities.
- Cellulite.
- Persistent feeling of heaviness in the legs.
- Constant sensation of cold feet.
- Impaired metabolism.
- Body intoxication.

Contraindications for Lymphatic Drainage Massage of the Legs

While lymphatic drainage foot massage is generally safe for most people, there are some conditions and situations where it should be avoided:

Absolute Contraindications

These conditions prohibit the use of lymphatic drainage massage under any circumstances:

- Blood, heart, and blood vessel diseases such as hemophilia, thrombosis, thrombophlebitis, heart valve defects, and acute myocardial ischemia.

- Renal, hepatic, pulmonary-heart failure.

- Serious mental illness.

- Pathologies of the lymphatic system.

- Diabetes.

- Active tuberculosis.

- Osteomyelitis (bone marrow inflammation).

- AIDS.

- Cancer, gangrene, and other severe pathologies.

Temporary Contraindications

These conditions temporarily prevent the use of lymphatic drainage massage until they are resolved or stabilized:

- Fever.

- Flu, cold, sore throat (ARVI).

- Acute inflammation and suppuration anywhere in the body.

- Exacerbations of chronic diseases.

- Inflammation of the lymph nodes.

- Nausea, vomiting, abdominal pain.

- Allergic skin rashes with hemorrhages.

- Hypertensive or hypotensive crisis.

- Abdominal organ diseases with bleeding risks.

- Venereal diseases.

Local Contraindications

These conditions impose restrictions only on the legs but may allow massage on unaffected parts of the body:

- Advanced varicose veins with significant bulging or lumps.

Before starting lymphatic drainage foot massage, consult with a healthcare professional to ensure it is safe for your specific health condition and needs.

Local Contraindications for Lymphatic Drainage Foot Massage

During a lymphatic drainage foot massage, certain areas should not be massaged due to specific conditions:

- Unhealed Wounds, Abrasions, Irritations: Avoid massaging over areas with open wounds, cuts, or skin irritations.

- Large and Protruding Moles, Nevi, Warts: Do not massage over prominent moles, birthmarks, or warts to avoid irritation or injury.

- Infectious and Fungal Skin Lesions: Areas affected by conditions like psoriasis, eczema, herpes, or fungal infections should not be massaged to prevent spreading or exacerbating the condition.

- Allergic Rashes: Avoid massaging over areas with allergic rashes to prevent further skin irritation.

- Varicose Veins Grade 3: Do not massage areas with advanced varicose veins where the veins are visibly bulging or have formed lumps.

Preparation for a Lymphatic Drainage Foot Massage

Before undergoing a lymphatic drainage foot massage, follow these preparation steps:

- Stay Hydrated: Drink at least 2 liters of water throughout the day to help disperse lymph and eliminate toxins. Have a glass of water immediately before the massage to maintain your body's water-salt balance.

- Warm Up: Take a hot shower or bath to warm up your body. Ideally, perform the massage right after bathing or using a sauna.

- Use of Products: Depending on the massage tools (vacuum cups or dry brush), apply oil or squalane to your feet and buttocks. Natural oils help the tools glide smoothly and provide additional benefits.

Chapter 6

Techniques for Performing Lymphatic Drainage Foot Massage at Home

Massage with Vacuum Cups

1. Preparation: Apply oil or squalane to your feet and buttocks for smooth gliding of the cups.

2. Massage Technique:

 - Begin at the ankles and move the largest cup upwards towards the pelvis, following the direction of lymph flow.

 - Avoid massaging the inner thighs and back of the knees.

- Move to the thighs, using the cup in upward and downward strokes.

- Once the tissue feels warmed up, switch to a smaller cup and massage the thighs in circular motions.

- Include the buttocks in circular massage movements.

3. Intensity: Don't shy away from firm and quick movements to stimulate circulation.

4. Duration: Massage each area for 7-10 minutes until the skin turns slightly red. Repeat every two days.

5. Expectations: Initially, you may experience bruising or discomfort, which should diminish as your body adapts to the massage.

Dry Brushing

- Use a dry brush in the bathroom to exfoliate dead skin cells without spreading them around the house.

- Brush from the feet upwards to the knees in rubbing movements, avoiding the back of the knees.

- Continue with the thighs and buttocks using circular motions.

By following these steps and techniques, you can effectively perform lymphatic drainage foot massage at home to enhance circulation, reduce swelling, and promote overall well-being. Always consult with a healthcare professional if you have specific health concerns or conditions before starting any massage therapy.

Chapter 7

Lymphatic Drainage Massage Techniques

Lymphatic drainage massage employs various techniques to benefit the body:

- Point (Projection) Technique: Targets specific areas near major lymph nodes using microcurrents and pressotherapy.

- Deep Technique: Applies pressure to muscle tissue using hand movements.

- Superficial Technique: Light fingertip movements on the skin's surface with gentle pressure.

Effects of the Procedure

Lymphatic drainage massage achieves positive changes by relaxing muscles around lymphatic vessels and increasing lymphatic flow speed:

- Mood Normalization
- Reduction in Fatigue, Improvement in Well-being
- Strengthening of Veins, Reduction of Varicose Veins
- Body Contouring, Cellulite Reduction
- Improved Skin Condition
- Reduction or Elimination of Edema
- General Weight Loss

Suitability of Lymphatic Drainage Massage

Determining the suitability of lymphatic drainage massage depends on consultation with a specialist, considering both indications and contraindications.

Indications

Lymphatic drainage massage is recommended for:

- Rehabilitation after injuries and surgeries
- Lymphedema (fluid retention)
- Poor psychological state
- Facial tissue sagging
- Decreased skin elasticity
- Early stages of varicose veins
- Scar and stretch mark improvement
- Slow skin healing
- Loss of skin tone and sagging

- Cellulite reduction
- Swelling, excess weight
- Slowed metabolism

Contraindications

Lymphatic drainage massage is not suitable for individuals with:

- Pregnancy
- Lymphadenopathy (enlarged lymph nodes)
- Heart and kidney failure
- Epilepsy
- Acute thrombophlebitis
- Benign tumors increasing in size
- Acute skin diseases
- Leg artery diseases causing ischemia
- Advanced varicose veins
- Oncological diseases

Differences and Advantages Over Other Massage Types

Lymphatic drainage massage differs significantly from classic and anti-cellulite massages:

- Targeted Areas and Fluid Direction: Focuses on lymph nodes and fluid flow direction.
- Varicose Vein Treatment: Addresses varicose veins effectively.
- Versatility and Painlessness: Can be applied to various conditions and is generally painless compared to other techniques.

Chapter 8

Benefits of Lymphatic Drainage

Lymphatic drainage offers numerous benefits for both physical and mental well-being. Doing lymphatic drainage yourself can be highly advantageous. Here are some of its key benefits:

- Detoxification: Helps eliminate toxins from the body, reducing water retention and promoting a lighter feeling.

- Immune System Support: Stimulates immune cell circulation, strengthening the body's defenses. Lymphocytes, immune cells found in lymph, travel more effectively to lymph nodes to fight pathogens.

- Digestive System Support: Promotes waste elimination, improving digestion and nutrient absorption. Helps alleviate constipation and bloating.

- Skin Improvement: Enhances skin appearance by reducing cellulite and stimulating cell renewal.

- Stress and Anxiety Reduction: Gentle massage promotes relaxation, calming the nervous system.

- Headache and Migraine Relief: Can alleviate tension and improve circulation in the head and neck, reducing headaches and migraines.

- Improved Sleep: Facilitates relaxation and stress reduction, potentially enhancing sleep quality.

- Enhanced Blood Circulation: Boosts lymph circulation, improving overall blood flow for better oxygen and nutrient delivery to tissues.

Chapter 9

How Lifestyle Affects the Lymphatic System

Several lifestyle factors significantly impact the health of the lymphatic system. Since the lymphatic system relies on body pressure to move lymph, activities that enhance efficiency include:

- Exercise: Increases blood flow, which in turn boosts lymph movement. This helps remove excess fluids and pathogens more efficiently.

- Hydration: Drinking plenty of water maintains lymphatic system health. Dehydration slows lymph circulation, leading to fluid accumulation and swelling in tissues.

- Limiting Caffeine and Alcohol: These substances dehydrate the body, hindering lymphatic circulation and contributing to fluid retention.

- Avoiding Toxins: Minimizing exposure to environmental toxins and unhealthy foods supports the lymphatic system's ability to protect the body from illness.

- Reducing Salt Intake: Salty foods cause fluid retention, challenging the lymphatic system's ability to remove excess fluids.

- Receiving Lymphatic Drainage Massages: These massages stimulate lymphatic flow, aiding efficient drainage of lymph from the body.

By incorporating these practices into daily life, individuals can support their lymphatic system's health and overall well-being effectively.

Chapter 10

After a Lymphatic Drainage Massage

After your lymphatic drainage massage, follow these steps to enhance its benefits and maintain its effects:

- Drink Plenty of Water: Your massage therapist has worked to stimulate lymph movement throughout your body. Drinking water after the massage helps to maximize these effects and supports ongoing detoxification.

- Eat Lightly: Opt for a light meal after your massage. While the massage strokes are gentle, they involve deep work. Give your body time to process this and avoid heavy meals that may overwhelm your digestive system.

- Engage in Light Exercise: Light physical activity, like gentle yoga, Pilates, or a short walk, helps maintain lymphatic circulation and enhances the detox process initiated by the massage. Avoid strenuous activities; focus on gentle movements that support relaxation and circulation.

- Get Adequate Rest: You may feel a bit tired after the massage, which is normal as your body focuses on detoxifying. Aim for a good night's sleep to support recovery and maximize the relaxing effects of the massage on your nervous system.

By following these steps, you can prolong the benefits of your lymphatic drainage massage and promote overall well-being effectively.

Chapter 11

Other Types of Massages Supporting Lymphatic Drainage

Miracle Sculpt

Miracle Sculpt combines the benefits of lymphatic drainage with shaping massage to offer a dual-purpose treatment. Unlike traditional lymphatic drainage massages that focus on reducing fluid retention, Miracle Sculpt adds a unique approach by targeting both excess liquids and stubborn fat deposits.

Described as a "manual liposculpture," Miracle Sculpt uses rhythmic suction and massaging strokes to drain excess fluids and break down fat. This technique not only reduces swelling but also contours the body, giving it a more defined shape. The massage strokes are gentle, ensuring comfort without causing pain or bruising.

While traditional shaping massages concentrate on specific areas like the buttocks, abdomen, and thighs, Miracle Sculpt provides a comprehensive whole-body approach. By enhancing lymphatic circulation, it helps the body process fat more efficiently, resulting in reduced puffiness, improved skin tone, and minimized cellulite appearance.

Velashape 3

Velashape 3 is a non-invasive treatment targeting fat cells and cellulite reduction. Using a handheld device, the treatment combines vacuum technology, infrared light, and radiofrequency to reshape the body. The vacuum and rollers loosen connective tissues, while the infrared light and radiofrequency shrink fat cells, leading to smoother skin and reduced circumference.

In addition to fat reduction, Velashape 3 stimulates lymphatic drainage by releasing fluids trapped in tissues. This process supports the body's natural detoxification and enhances the results of fat reduction treatments. Each session lasts about 30 minutes with no downtime, making it a convenient option for those seeking body contouring.

Combining Velashape 3 with lymphatic drainage massages like Miracle Sculpt further accelerates fat elimination and fluid drainage. By optimizing the lymphatic system's function, these treatments help achieve more pronounced weight loss and a slimmer body shape over time.

Chapter 12

Contraindications to Lymphatic Drainage

Lymphatic drainage, like any therapy, has certain conditions where caution is advised to prevent complications or health risks. These include:

- Thrombosis (blood clotting)
- Phlebitis (vein inflammation)
- Tuberculosis
- Heart problems
- Hypertension (high blood pressure)
- Cancer, cysts, untreated tumors
- Hyperthyroidism
- Asthma

- Infectious skin diseases

If you have any doubts about whether lymphatic drainage is suitable for you, it's crucial to consult your doctor for personalized advice. Some conditions may require medication or antibiotics that could interfere with lymphatic drainage treatments.

It's also advisable to avoid lymphatic drainage during fever or active inflammation to prevent potential complications. Focusing on specific areas directly connected to the lymphatic system, such as the neck and ears, can sometimes be a safer alternative.

For effective lymphatic drainage, gentle and light movements are preferred because the lymphatic vessels are near the skin's surface.

The goal is not to apply pressure like reflexology or acupressure but rather to gently stimulate lymph flow towards the heart through pumping motions.

Syncing these movements with your breathing enhances their effectiveness and promotes mindfulness during the massage. Facial lymphatic drainage, in particular, offers detoxifying benefits and supports overall skin health. The lymphatic system helps regulate fluid balance, detoxify tissues, and boost immune function by producing white blood cells in lymph nodes.

Unlike the blood circulation system, which is aided by the heart's pumping action, the lymphatic system relies on breathing and muscle movement for circulation. This can sometimes be insufficient, especially during periods of inactivity.

By promoting lymphatic circulation through massage, you can enhance both beauty and well-being. Key benefits for the skin include reducing puffiness, inflammation, redness, and enhancing skin radiance.

Conclusion

Lymphatic drainage massage is gaining popularity for its health benefits and ability to reduce bloating and puffiness through gentle, relaxing techniques. Alongside traditional lymphatic drainage, newer methods like Miracle Sculpt and VelaShape 3 offer enhanced benefits in fluid elimination and fat reduction, making them sought-after treatments in spas worldwide.

Made in United States
Troutdale, OR
09/07/2024